POETRY
&
THE DISCOVERY OF MEDICINES

WILLIAM C. CAMPBELL

Published 2026 by Linguaphile Press. Hamilton, Virginia, USA

CONTENTS

INTRODUCTION

If variety is truly the spice of life, the following essays on two very different topics may be indicative of a fair amount of seasoning in my professional life.

In writing these essays I hope to retain the traditional distinction between essays and other types of literary article. The essay is advocacy, but not propaganda. It makes no claim to be evenhanded.

Until recently, it did not even occur to me that there is another reason for the appeal of the essay format. The word essay is both noun and verb and claiming to have made an attempt to have done something seems less brash than claiming to have done it.

I close this Introduction with three brief updates of previous writings:

- Those of us who write essays to vent opinions on a subject of special interest are likely to have minor interests that could hardly justify the writing of an essay but might warrant inclusion in a brief appendix. I have written elsewhere about the need for rehearsal in the telling of short stories. Clearly this applies to the public, not conversational, telling of stories.
- In previously offering guidelines for the introduction of the speakers on public occasions I suggested only proscription, giving the impression that public introduction (on college campuses, for example) must be somber affairs. In fact, such occasions are usually splendid opportunities for anecdotes and humorous remarks.

- The practical advantage of macrocyclic lactone anthelmintics in the control and prevention of heartworm disease in dogs rests largely on the fact that there are properties of those drugs that allow treatment to be given only once a month. It is sometimes assumed that this development was made possible by the efficacy of the drug against immature worms that have entered the host dog in the month or following treatment. In fact, however, the once-a-month treatment was effective because it was active against immature worms that had entered the dog body in the month or two prior to treatment. This illustrates the benefit of using mechanism-blind assay protocols in drug screening, and is of central importance in the field of drug discovery.

Poetry

Poetry, What's That? – A Scientist's 'Take' on Poetry

Why do you write poetry? There is a good chance that you don't. There is also a good chance that you have written poetry at some time in your life, and a very good chance that you have at least thought about doing it. I confess that I have written some of it myself; but now that I am old, I am trying to be brave and not do it anymore.

But why would *anybody* 'do' poetry . . . and what is it anyway?

Snappy descriptors of it seem to be everywhere, and I quote a few in the paragraphs that follow. Whether they be witty, dumb, humorous, insightful, or whatever, they might tell us something about poetry, but they don't tell us what it actually is. For that, we need a definition, and definitions tend to be held in custody in dictionaries. Having thus trapped myself into practicing what I am in danger of preaching, I admit that I have had the effrontery to cobble together my own 'working definition':

> *Poetry is a branch of literature in which an author uses extraordinary language to record or evoke feelings or thoughts that the author deems sufficiently surprising or original to warrant sharing with others.*

That may be a bit more elaborate than other definitions, but I believe it will be found fundamentally in accord with definitions that appear in ordinary respectable dictionaries. Sometimes 'evoking' an emotion involves awakening it from slumber, which aligns well with landscape painter George Inness's saying that the goal of any artwork is to "awaken" an emotion.

It used to be (especially in the 1980s) that if I happened to think of something unusual and intriguing, I would record it on paper in some rough form, and that form would be a sort of poetry, more or less. I think I did that because I wondered if anyone else had had the same thought. If so, the experience would constitute a sort of kinship, an entirely imaginary kinship!

Most likely, of course, I would never know whether or not my thought had already been thought! But perhaps I could still share my thoughts with others by putting them into a poem. Writing poems, I suppose, can almost be part of the give-and-take of 'the kindness of strangers.'

The thought that triggers a poem does not have to be profound, and for most of us, there is comfort in that. For me, however, the inciting thought does have to be surprising. In the 18th century, Wordsworth wrote of poetry as the "spontaneous overflow of powerful feeling". I find the element of surprise more important than the element of intensity (of being "powerful"). 'Surprise' implies that the author has not had quite the same feelings or thoughts in the past, and it is their novelty that generates a desire to share them with others. It is a desire borne, perhaps, from a hope that feelings can be validated by knowing that others have them, too.

I didn't think about any of that stuff back when I was writing poems. There was no deliberate analysis of a motivational process on my part. There was, I guess, some reflection on the subject of the poem, but no wandering through philosophical mazes in search of a reason for writing. It is only in retrospect that I am now trying to put into words the genesis of a poetry-writing impulse that was with me for a considerable part of my life.

In the mid-1980s, in a what-the-heck mood, I sent two poems to the journal *Perspectives in Biology and Medicine*, published by the University of Chicago Press. To my satisfaction and astonishment, the poems appeared in widely separated pages of the autumn issue of 1987. Such acceptance is likely, unless one is of an Emily-Dickinson sort of temperament, to result in further dispatches to editorial desks. I continued to send poems to *Perspectives* until it was no longer published by the University of Chicago Press (and was no longer publishing poetry).

So, *someone* thought some of my 'poems' were indeed poems. Were they right? Is there a proper way to tell? Harking back to the beginning of this rumination, we could be unfashionable and consult our dictionaries. Alternatively, we could look for illumination in the words of the "greats." WH Auden said, "Of the many definitions of poetry, the simplest is still the best: 'memorable speech.' Surely, he should be held accountable for (apparently) not looking up the definition of 'definition' in his dictionary!

One might sense the longing of Emily Dickinson in writing "To see the Summer Sky Is Poetry, though never in a book it lie . . ." but again one must protest! What happened to literature? . . . not even a handwritten scribble? Is an alphabet of letters no longer needed? What, indeed, happened to art, now stripped of its requirement for artifice? Those who find poetry everywhere will discover that there is no poetry anywhere. A sad thought.

THE LITERARY COMPOSITION OF POEMS

You may have trouble deciding whether to write your poem in "free verse" or within one of the many established forms of structured and rhymed verse. If so, you are in good company. This tension between freedom and form has long occupied poets and critics alike. Personally, I have found value in both approaches: the openness of free verse offers flexibility of thought and expression, while formal structures impose a discipline that can sharpen language and intensify meaning.

The oft-quoted remark by Robert Frost, that writing free verse is like playing tennis without a net, captures a skepticism toward the absence of constraint. Yet the remark is not without irony, as many of Frost's own most celebrated poems depart from strict formal limitations. This suggests that even those who advocate structure recognize the creative possibilities that arise when rules are bent or selectively ignored.

A similar ambivalence can be observed in the work of John Milton who used rhyme and an entirely conventional form of sonnet for *On His Blindness*, but only a few years later, justified his use of 'blank verse' for Paradise Lost, saying that he was rejecting the "troublesome and modern bondage of rhyming" which had been "the invention of a barbarous age." [Archambeau, Robert. Inventions of a Barbarous Age: Contemporary Rhyme in Poetry. Spoon River Poetry Review Issue 39.2: www.srpr.org] Milton's position reflects a broader historical pattern in which poetic form evolves not through rejection alone, but through redefinition.

On the Subject of the Subject

Many people would agree that the surest way to ruin a perfectly good poem is to explain it. There is a good deal of truth in that view, but only up to a point. Explanation, when it becomes reductive or overly directive, can strip a poem of its suggestiveness and diminish the reader's opportunity for discovery. Yet the complete rejection of explanation may be equally problematic, particularly in the context of much contemporary poetry, where obscurity can sometimes impede rather than enrich understanding.

It is often said, sometimes with a hint of resignation, that modern poetry is "over one's head." I am not entirely unsympathetic to that sentiment. However, difficulty in itself is not a fault. Higher mathematics, for example, is also beyond the grasp of most readers, yet mathematicians do not routinely present their most complex formulations without some form of interpretive framework. There is, in other words, an implicit acknowledgment that complexity benefits from mediation. Poetry, especially when it draws upon specialized knowledge, cultural references, or unconventional structures, may similarly require a degree of contextual support if it is to achieve its full effect.

This does not imply that a poem must be accompanied by a formal exegesis, nor that its meaning should be fixed in advance. Rather, it suggests that there exists a spectrum between complete opacity and excessive explanation. The appropriate position on that spectrum will vary depending on the nature of the poem and the background of its intended audience. A poem grounded in widely shared experiences may require little or no elaboration, whereas one that engages with more specialized domains, such as science or history, may benefit from a modest degree of clarification.

In my own case, many poems have been written with readers in mind who possess some familiarity with scientific or historical themes. Even so, it has always been my hope that they might resonate beyond that immediate circle. If a brief explanation can serve as a bridge, without constraining interpretation, then it may enhance rather than diminish the poem's capacity to engage.

THE NATURE OF POETRY

Further thoughts on the nature of poetry which I share below, were developed when I was invited to contribute a Foreword for a book of photographs and poems by Irish surgeon Michael Sugrue. [Donegal's Atlantic Way, 2019, ISBN 978-1913069-15-5].

"Science and art are profoundly different, but they have always been compatible bedfellows. Practitioners of both are driven by an urge to do, or to create, something new. One strives for objectivity, the other revels in the subjective, but creativity is the hallmark of both. This holds true, more narrowly, for medicine and literature.

"Contemporaries of the great 18th-century physician-philosopher Erasmus Darwin considered him one of the greatest poets of his era.

Modern readers, struggling through one of his long poems, will shake their heads in disbelief at such an assessment, but poetry evolves through taste and tradition. Medicine tries to hold those elements subordinate to fact, hypothesis, and reasoned probability, but science, too, is subject to perpetual challenge and change.

Erasmus Darwin is largely forgotten today (except as someone else's grandfather), but his accomplishments at desk and bedside live on in history, glittering flotsam in the stream of knowledge that has no end. Medicos as far apart in place and time as Anton Chekov and William Carlos Williams have also trodden dual pathways, leading relatively quiet lives as family doctors while at the same time pursuing their literary passion with great, and durable, success.

"Archibald McLeish famously said that a poem does not have to mean anything but has to simply "be." Though tucked into a poem, that remark is widely and approvingly quoted. I used to think that it was usefully provocative, but the more it provoked me to think, the more I thought that it was singularly unhelpful. A poem cannot exist in a vacuum. A poem must reach the consciousness of a reader or listener, must say something even if no one is listening. The reader may not 'hear,' and the poet may not care about that. The poem may proffer profundity; it may proffer puzzlement; it may entertain; it may show off technical virtuosity in a display of verbal fireworks. It is what is proffered that makes the poem. It is by our reception of it and response to it that we should judge it.

Will there be resonance... or empty rattle?

"A pithy remark that is more to my liking is Robert Frost's comment that 'poetry is language that says more.' It is tempting to ask 'more of what?' but, deep down, we suspect that the remark is perfect as it is. Good poetry has a good deal of mystery about it.

"Much of today's poetry gives me a sense of unease. Should one even wonder what the poems are about? Does the question itself expose a lack of cultural awareness? Naïve or not, I am driven toward the conclusion that Frost's remark is turned on its head by many of today's poems, in which poetry seems to be language that says less. Of interest in this context is a response from one famous physicist to another.

Robert Oppenheimer had remarked to Paul Dirac that, were he not a physicist, he would want to be a poet. Dirac's reaction was utter bafflement. It was his understanding that the objective of the physicist was to take something obscure and make it clear, whereas the purpose of the poet was exactly the opposite. I think there is more than a hint of truth in Dirac's point of view, but his puzzlement is more striking than his pronouncement. There is nothing baffling about Oppenheimer's wistfulness!

A half-century ago, Will Cuppy, while poking fun at the obscurity that is so often a feature of modern poetry, warned that "those who wish to communicate with me by means of the written word must do so in prose." He may have been writing as a humorist, but I think there is a deeper insight to be found in his words. As mentioned above, I think of poetry as an open-handed 'proffering' of thought or emotion, something quite distinct from communication of information directed toward a specific individual or toward a generalized audience or readership. The first case might be likened to a placing of delicacies on a table of infinite scope with an implied invitation for passers-by to help themselves as they wished. Communication, on the other hand, seems more akin to presenting nourishment to people with an expectation, or at least a hope, that it would be consumed. It is a duality that, like poetry itself, does not lend itself to rigorous intellectual debate.

Poetry has indeed been used to communicate information. In ancient times, rhetorical poetry with versification and rhyming undoubtedly facilitated the perpetuation of oral history and tribal culture. That, however, seems far removed from poetry as we know it today.

The Persona Conundrum

Many years ago, a friend sent me one of his poems, a poem with a first-person account of a heroic battlefield episode in wartime. I was greatly touched by my friend's words, and told him that I had not known of his military service and combat experience. He, a professional lexicographer, quickly assured me that he had no such experience and that his poem had expressed the thoughts of the poem's 'persona'. Being then unaware of the 'persona' concept, I felt that I had been misled by my friend. I was later to find out that such a concept was widely recognized, and that there was some history of intellectual agonizing over the significance of poetry written in the first-person singular, particularly as to whether the "I" of the poem represents the poet, or represents someone else, the "persona" or 'speaker.'

In fields of endeavor marked by vague boundaries rather than strict rules, it can be helpful to adopt a 'working operational system' where some level of arbitrariness is acceptable. For me, I mainly rely on the 'persona' concept when I want to write on behalf of someone or something, but feel it would be presumptuous to do so directly due to my lack of firsthand knowledge. This approach will be reflected in the poems *'Smallpox Maiden', 'Suppose', 'Villanelle for a Small Victim of AIDS', and 'The Lesser Circulation'.*

In a setting from the distant past, there's usually no need to explicitly acknowledge the Persona in a poem or even consider the Persona concept. If my poem attributes thoughts to a long-deceased person, those thoughts should be genuine in the sense that I believe my words would mirror what that person might have thought if expressed by them. There might be instances where it is hard to distinguish the poet from the poem, but in any case, avoiding deception must remain the primary rule. There are, however, occasions when I write a poem that is unashamedly autobiographical. Whether a reader realizes it or not, I want the Persona to be me. That would apply to the poems '*I Know You Cannot Hear Me*', '*Hiroshima*', and *'I Will Climb the Hill Beyond Cloonmas'*....

A CLOSING WORD TO THE WISE

William Wordsworth did not become one of literature's "immortals" merely by feeling his heart stir at the sight of a rainbow, nor by privately refining that feeling into a more mature or sophisticated metaphor. What distinguishes him, and, indeed, any enduring poet, is the act of committing that experience to language. The fleeting moment of perception, however vivid, acquires permanence and communicative power only when it is shaped, articulated, and shared.

In this sense, poetry is not simply a matter of feeling or even of insight; it is an act of deliberate expression. The unwritten poem, however profound in conception, remains inert. It is through the discipline of writing that thought is clarified, emotion is given form, and experience becomes accessible to others. To write, then, is not merely to record; it is to transform. And it is in that transformation that poetry secures its place, not only in literature, but in the continuing dialogue of human understanding.

HIROSHIMA EVENING

Were you here, old man, were you
anywhere near?

Stooped and alone, you shuffle along,
soft step on the concrete,
steadfastly slipping past
the neon lights of a hamburger stand,
into the endless dark.

Come back, old man! I still want to know.
Did you wake from young dreams?
In this place? Were you here?
Were you anywhere near
When it happened?

Or were you on an earlier night?
crouched above a far-off sea,
elated and trembling, and
hurtling full-throttle toward
another history?

WILLIAM C. CAMPBELL

Perspectives in Biology and Medicine, 35, 3, page 338.
Spring 1992

You Cannot Hear Me

I know you cannot hear me now.
Your head lies absolutely still
upon the pillow.
Magically,
you slip away from all your years.
Funny to think that those dry lips
once crooned away my infant cry,
and that those wrinkled remnant arms
held me aloft so we might shout!
I'm glad the nurse has left the room.
(Insane but true that I should care!)
For I must say aloud those words
I dared not say when I was young
and did not say in later years
because my life was far away;
(Although in truth, I know that I
would not have said them anyhow.)
It's too late now, and yet, dear God
make of these words a laser beam
that they might breach the walls of that
insensate ear and find their mark.
One moment more before I leave
alone, alone with you, I grieve.

W. C. CAMPBELL

Perspectives in Biology and Medicine, 32, 2, page 271.
Winter 1989.

THE DISCOVERY OF MEDICINES

THESIS ON

RESEARCH TOWARD DISCOVERY AND DEVELOPMENT OF NOVEL MEDICINES

1. INTRODUCTION: A THWARTED THESIS AND A COSTLY NEGLECT OF SCIENTIFIC PRINCIPLE

For the past half-century, I have advanced a specific thesis concerning the principles of new drug discovery. It is applicable to various categories of metazoan pathogens, but is particularly applicable to diseases caused by bacterial and helminthic (worm) pathogens. While viruses and prions continue to occupy a bizarre spot in the universe of Life, this discourse does not concern them. The main points of the thesis can be summarized succinctly:

1. Throughout history, two main approaches have been taken to the discovery of new drugs:
    a. *Finding* them, by chance or through trial-and-error experimentation; widely known as the EMPIRICAL APPROACH.
    b. *Creating*, devising, or designing them on the basis of scientific research on the fundamental nature of the pathogen and its relationship to its host; widely known as the RATIONAL APPROACH.

c. For BOTH approaches, it is understood that 'discovery' refers to the detection of a 'lead compound,' a substance that has, to some degree, the desired anti-pathogen and non-biocidal characteristics, and thus has to some evident degree, the potential of being developed into a useful medication.

d. Throughout history, the number of useful drugs discovered by the Empirical Method has far exceeded the number discovered by the Rational Method.

e. In the 21st century, the Empirical Method has largely been discarded by the biomedical community (academic, industrial, institutional) in favor of the Rational Method. The widespread rejection of empiricism is difficult to justify on rational grounds and results in harmful neglect of social responsibility.

For ages, medicinal stuff, 'Materia Medica' in its Latin guise, was an essential subject of study in medical education. Its content was primarily herbal, though a few mineral and animal items were included. Its books and its mentors were filled with botanical learning. The term was in use at least as far back as the 1st century, when Dioscorides wrote his phenomenally influential five-volume treatise "de Materia Medica." For the purposes of the discussion here, know that I am concerned with the physical matter of medication.

Although it is customary to acknowledge the contributions of ancient thinkers, such discussion falls outside the scope of this work. Early scientific observations, while often accurate, were deeply intertwined with myth and mysticism. For clarity and relevance, these historical antecedents are set aside in favor of focusing on modern scientific approaches.

My working definition of science is: The orderly assemblage, pursuit, and propagation of evidence-based knowledge. My purpose is to call attention to a benefit of science that is extremely important but widely and needlessly neglected.

Although science has been misused in harmful ways, such instances are widely condemned. In contrast, its application in ethical drug discovery is broadly regarded as beneficial. It is within this context that scientific effort should serve clear medical and societal value. It is in the context of this endeavor, new drug discovery, that I level a charge of neglect.

2. OPERATIONAL OUTLINE

The operational mode of the Rational Approach is sufficiently evident from its definition in item B, above.

The operational mode of the Empirical Approach can be stated simply as: the testing of a variety of substances for signs of efficacy against the target pathogen, keeping in mind that:

a) The greater the number of substances tested, the greater the probability of success.

b) The greater the variety of substances tested, the greater the probability of success. The testing of substances chosen on the basis of perceived likelihood of success is acceptable and has no downside other than the possible wasting of 'test slots' when resources are limited.

c) Test substances should be apportioned in such a way that there will be sufficient material to allow confirmatory tests in the event that 'activity' (evidence of efficacy, however slight) is recorded.

In the context of drug discovery, the empirical approach has become only marginally acceptable.

3. THE HEART OF THE PROBLEM

One would expect humankind to feel a moral or public-health obligation to limit the harm caused by infectious disease. Given alternative approaches, the logic of science suggests greater consideration should be given to methods with a strong record of success rather than those with little success. It seems axiomatic that an approach with a greater probability of success should not be subordinated to one with a lesser probability. The discovery of sulfa drugs in the 19th century justified expanded industrial screening of related compounds, later giving way to "random" screening. Since novelty is crucial in medicinal products, it is advantageous to screen substances regardless of known or suspected biochemical properties.

The value of mechanism-based 'Rational 'research on drugs is not in doubt, but that should not distract us from the present issue of the success-probability of a particular approach. It is largely up to the managers and directors of scientific projects to guide the choice of approach. If they believe in the value of empirical screening, they will accept the financial, managerial, and psychological challenges of such work.

There is, however, yet another aspect that needs consideration. If, as I believe to be the case, failure to undertake empirical screening results in failure to discover valuable drugs, then there is an ethical component to the discussion. Do scientists have a moral right to continue to neglect the Empirical Approach?

4. FURTHERMORE

These reflections are presented entirely in the context of microbial diseases, specifically those caused by bacterial, protozoan, and helminthic parasites. They are not intended to apply to degenerative or metabolic diseases, nor to viral diseases, as viruses occupy a distinct niche and differ fundamentally from other pathogens. Although there is a widespread global effort to apply science in many ways, the focus here is on the egregious neglect of a particular use of science in addressing these microbial diseases.

Paracelsus warned his readers "not to reject the message of experiment." He added: "For every experiment is like a weapon which must be used according to its peculiar power, as a spear to thrust, a club to strike, so also is it with experiments." (Jaffe, 2012)

Our reputable universities are assumed to be highlights of civilized society, but there are also shortcomings that may be less widely recognized.

Some recent scholarly analysis has alleged that university research has a particular relevant shortcoming: The process of generating knowledge through research has not paid adequate attention to the social impact of its outcomes. (Crow, M. M., & Dabars, W. B., 2020).

The undervaluing of empirical research is not limited to helminth or ectoparasite studies, nor to infections. It applies to any condition where a suitable bioassay exists. Once a key disease marker is identified, it should be considered as the basis for a high-throughput assay to support empirical investigation.

In the pursuit of scientific discovery, cultural influences and psychological quirks can be calamitous if not recognized. It has long seemed to me that many drug researchers become entrapped in viewing the empirical approach as intrinsically inferior to the rational, thereby belittling mechanism-blind ("random") screening. One might think that the approach leading to thiabendazole, levamisole, and ivermectin could yield further useful agents, but this insight is often ignored. We may never know how many valuable drugs were missed due to this subtle scientific arrogance.

Some bright spots can be discerned in the intellectual gloom of drug non-discovery. One is the creation of novel managerial strategies, such as DARPA, which brought unprecedented interdisciplinary depth, though focused mainly on antiviral treatment and not on the empirical-rational distinction. That distinction, however, does appear in and is essential to another example: Dr. Jo Handelsman's work, which demonstrates that even mechanism-blind screening can serve as a powerful tool for teaching microbiological skills while yielding novel compounds and revealing previously unknown biodynamic processes.

The possible role of "bias" in the demise of empiricism in drug discovery is introduced here because the change in research strategy (from Empirical to Rational) does not seem to be merely a matter of professional fashion but rather a matter of intellectual respectability. Indeed, the situation remains as depressing as I saw it some years ago: The trouble with the Empirical Approach is that it is intellectually disreputable no matter how successful. The trouble with the Rational Approach is that it is intellectually irresistible, no matter how unfruitful it has been, a tendency reflected in the historical prioritization of target-based strategies over phenotypic screening despite the latter's demonstrated productivity (Moffat et al., 2014).

5. GETTING LOST ON THE ROAD TO DISCOVERY

From the 1930s onward, it became traditional for the screening of chemicals for the detection of biodynamic compounds to be done primarily by the pharmaceutical industry. Perhaps the academic biomedical community would have been wise to recognize that industrial corporations found it more useful in the long-run to discover effective (and profitable) drugs by finding them than to attempt to devise them (no matter how brilliantly) on theoretical grounds. By the beginning of the 21st century, the tradition had changed. The ranks of industrial scientists became populated with recently-trained scientists, understandably eager to participate in the excitement and the rewards of the molecular revolution in biology, and to contribute to the sensational discoveries being made almost daily (in vaccines against viral diseases, for example). Exploiting chance through random screening was not appealing; the Rational Approach to drug discovery is now standard in most academic and industrial laboratories.

Since that is not likely to change anytime soon, I have pointed to a new way to reap the benefit of empirical drug discovery, but its implementation would face many logistical and managerial difficulties (Kiriiri, G. K et al., 2020).

In ordinary circumstances, it is supposed that a broad target is easier to hit than a narrow one. A Rational drug exploration is usually focused on a relatively specific chemical substance or biochemical pathway. Empirical screening, on the other hand, deals with multiple targets, each one being hypothetical, thus of unknown structure. In this endeavor, the key to success lies not in the width of a target, but in the number of bioactive compounds (targets) that might be isolated from whatever number of test substances a given assay system can handle.

There is nothing freakish about such empiricism. I would be reluctant to consider it a matter of subconscious bias. It is a matter of probability. It is logical. It is scientific. And time and again it has worked. Why then has it fallen into disrepute and neglect? I know of no satisfactory explanation, and am driven to the unhappy suspicion that it is a matter of subconscious bias on the part of the biomedical community, and especially the would-be drug discoverers among them.

In the last two decades of the 20th century, there was a marked falling off in the introduction of new agents for controlling bacterial and parasitic diseases (Silver, L. L. 2011). The trend has persisted up to the present, and much concern is being expressed about the clinical consequences, especially in the face of widespread resistance against many of the current medications. In the context of seeking an explanation for this shortage of new antimicrobial drugs, I find it compelling to associate the shortage of drugs with the abandonment of the Empirical Approach to drug discovery.

Admittedly, the concept of empiricism can be pushed to a point at which it seems absurd, almost unscientific. For example, the essay that enabled the discovery of the anthelmintic ivermectin can be reduced to the following brief recipe: Take a batch of worm-infected mice. Supplement the diet of each mouse for a period of one week with an unknown amount of an unknown substance that might not be there. Wait another week. Examine each mouse to determine if it is still infected with the worms. Absence of worms is recorded as apparent evidence of the presence of a biodynamic substance. Thus, this successful assay may be described in a way that makes it seem like a parody of science while yet conforming to the essential elements of the enterprise.

6. THE OUTCOME: ARGUMENT FROM THE OTHER SIDE

Unaccountably, others have not lined up to lend support to my appeal for reconsideration of the empirical approach.

A few individuals have glibly offered verbal support while proceeding to ignore its implications. I have come to the conclusion that its failure is rooted more in psychology than in laboratory science. That presents aw formidable impasse.

How do the experts react to the dilemma I have outlined? They resort to a most curious suspension of scientific logic. If you pay attention to the relevant lay and professional literature, you will see examples. One eminent expert recently published an article to alert the public to the acute global need for the discovery of new antimicrobial drugs through a rational approach. A very small personal poll of scientific experts suggests that few, if any, shared my outrage at this statement. Why was the public not simply alerted to the need for new antimicrobial drugs? What possessed the expert to specify the need for drugs discovered by only one of the two classical approaches? and to pick the method that has consistently failed!?

The common, but unacknowledged, bias against empiricism was evident during the ivermectin-as-treatment-for-COVID-19 controversy. Eminent scientists have demanded experimental evidence (or at least a convincing theoretical postulate) of a biochemical mode of action in order to accept (theoretically) the antiparasitic agent as efficacious. That is to say, they set two absolute requirements for efficacy:

(a) strong clinical evidence of efficacy, and

(b) a creditable mode of action to account for the clinical efficacy.

The first item is indeed necessary; the second is highly desirable but is not a scientific requirement.

My bafflement here is not the occasional sloppy thinking (we all have our moments of sloppiness). But what causes an eminent expert to think sloppily even in composing a statement with evident deliberation? Could it be that rigorous thinking becomes subverted by an underlying bias, a widely shared bias, but one so committed to the rational approach that the empirical approach is simply forgotten? The underlying problem, in short, may well be a psychological one.

There remains a curious aspect of this whole "approach" scene. Occasionally, members of the 'rational' camp (the 'opposition') have declared themselves to be sympathizers with the 'empirical' point of view. All of them have been biochemists working on projects devoted to the discovery of anti-parasitic drugs. They were few in number and are in no way representative of the biochemical confraternity. Professionals as varied as a government researcher, a university professor from a well-regarded institution, an international pharmaceutical scientist, and others have mentioned they agree that the probability of near-time success is greater for the empirical 'screening' approach than for the 'rational' approach, but that they dared not say it openly lest their candor prove harmful to their career or to their professional reputation. They chose to confide in me, and I have been grateful for the honor. Their comments may not have been particularly valiant, but they were undoubtedly sincere.

Hundreds of antibacterial and antiparasitic agents have been discovered empirically, historically by capitalizing on folklore, with confirmation by clinical experience and testing, followed in time by natural-product isolation and standardization. With the flowering of chemical synthesis at the beginning of the 20th century, a new era was ushered in, and new drugs were discovered more and more by screening chemical compounds (and eventually natural products) for evidence of efficacy. We discovered, in short, how to discover such agents unpredictably by relying on chance occurrence.

In contrast, it is difficult to identify examples of the discovery of antibacterial or antiparasitic agents by the Rational Approach. Undoubtedly, many will rush to challenge so bold an assertion, and to mollify personal outrage by pointing out contradictions and exceptions.

They may, for example, point to the work of Hitchings and Elion, the rightly celebrated discoverers of Daraprim and related agents. But George Hitchings himself said that their work was firmly rooted in the earlier elucidation of the mode of action of the sulfur drugs (which were discovered empirically). That is relevant to the present discussion and is supportive of the underlying thesis, but in no way detracts from the brilliance of the rational component of the Hitchings-Elion discovery. Their work can be seen as an example of 'semi-rational drug discovery'. It is not, however, a good example, because of the disproportionately large rational component. A simpler and more instructive example would be the discovery of ethopabate $C_{12}H_{15}NO_4$ as a poultry coccidiostat.

Despite its historical success, the empirical method is subject to a practical constraint arising from a laudable human concern for the welfare and rights of animals used in research. One objective of a campaign to protect those rights was the design of experimental protocols that would minimize the number of animals used. The introduction of a one-animal per experimental group (Ostlind, et al. 2012) can be seen as one natural endpoint of that endeavor. As classical drug screening becomes more complex and expensive, it may become replaced by isolated components of animal life (cell culture, organoids and such), as platforms for primary screening. Care must, of course, be taken to preserve the mechanism-blind aspect of such assays.

I have reluctantly raised the possibility that the decline of empiricism in drug discovery might be a matter of "bias." It does not seem to be merely a matter of professional fashion but rather a matter of intellectual respectability. Indeed, the situation is as depressing as I saw it some years ago(J. Nematol. 15: 608-615, 1983): The trouble with the Empirical Approach is that it is intellectually disreputable no matter how successful. The trouble with the Rational Approach is that it is intellectually irresistible, no matter how unfruitful it has been.

REFERENCES

Crow, M. M., & Dabars, W. B. (2020). The fifth wave: The evolution of American higher education. Johns Hopkins University Press. https://issues.org/the-future-of-american-higher-education-crow-dabars-fifth-wave/

Jaffe, Bernard. (2012) Crucibles; Newton Publishing Company, New York, NY

Kiriiri, G. K., Njogu, P. M., & Mwangi, A. N. (2020). Exploring different approaches to improve the success of drug discovery and development projects: a review. Future Journal of Pharmaceutical Sciences, 6(1), 27. https://link.springer.com/article/10.1186/s43094-020-00047-9

Moffat, J. G., Rudolph, J., & Bailey, D. (2014). Phenotypic screening in cancer drug discovery—past, present and future. Nature reviews Drug discovery, 13(8), 588-602. https://www.nature.com/articles/nrd4366

Ostlind, Dan A. et al. "Efficacy of Ivermectin versus Dual Infections of Haemonchus Contortus and Heligmosomoides Polygyrus in the Mouse." The Journal of Parasitology, U.S. National Library of Medicine, 12 Nov. 2012, https://pubmed.ncbi.nlm.nih.gov/23145469/

Silver, L. L. (2011). Challenges of antibacterial discovery. Clinical microbiology reviews, 24(1), 71-109. https://journals.asm.org/doi/abs/10.1128/cmr.00030-10

www.ingramcontent.com/pod-product-compliance
Lightning Source LLC
LaVergne TN
LVHW011539110826
845483LV00005B/90
* 9 7 9 8 2 3 4 1 3 9 9 5 5 *